My Grief Diary

A WORKBOOK THROUGH GRIEF

A companion guide & confidante
through the aftermath of
heartbreaking loss

LYNDA CHELDELIN FELL
ANGIE CARTWRIGHT

Lynda Cheldelin Fell/AlyBlue Media
Ferndale, WA 98248
www.AlyBlueMedia.com
PRINTED IN THE U.S.A.

Cover Design by AlyBlue Media

My Grief Diary -- 1st ed.
Lynda Cheldelin Fell/Angie Cartwright
ISBN: 978-1-944328-10-8

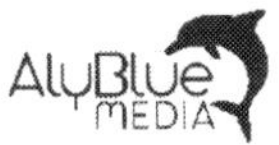

DEDICATION

In loving memory of
Rhonda Sue Newsome
Alyssa Victoria Yvonne Fell.

Walking with a friend in the dark
is better than walking alone in the light.

HELEN KELLER

CONTENTS

Strength is being your truest self.
No matter what anyone else thinks.

ANGIE CARTWRIGHT

ABOUT THIS WORKBOOK

Grief is a long, hard journey that is as unique to each griever as one's fingerprint. While there is no single "cure" for grief, there are numerous tools that offer comfort and encouragement along your journey. And *My Grief Diary* is designed to be one of these tools.

Broken into two parts, this workbook allows you to express your grief in a safe and comforting manner, like you're among friends. And you are, for we compiled this workbook from our hearts to yours.... hearts of grievers uniting in our grief. The first part offers assignments designed to help you face your grief. The second part offers assignments to help you learn how to live again as you reassemble the pieces. Throughout you will find personal, candid reflections from both of us.

Healing is a collaborative effort between yourself, your family and friends, your healthcare providers, and even us. We encourage you to share the assignments with your doctor, counselor, and/or therapist. As healing is not a process to be rushed, neither is your completion of this workbook. In fact, we encourage you to take your time with each assignment, possibly days and even weeks. There is nothing to be gained by rushing, and everything to be gained by taking your time.

Please note that we use the word "heal." That is an important concept to keep close to your heart. Grief turns one's life upside down, shreds it to pieces. And healing takes time and, well let's face it, we have nothing but time in the aftermath of loss. Maybe your life will never be the same as it was, but with hard work, lots of patience, and tender loving care of yourself, you can find your footing once again and even feel moments of peace and joy. We are living proof of that.

Please use us as your inspiration whenever the waves of grief wash over you, let us be your umbrella during the moments of torrential downpour. We have walked and survived the storms of grief to find that peace, and even joy, do indeed exist in the aftermath. We know you can do it too, and we want to help. In fact, we'll be your biggest cheerleaders, so don't give up! We are here every step of the way.

From our hearts to your heart,

Lynda Cheldelin Fell
& Angie Cartwright

Hugs are and always will be
better than words.

LYNDA CHELDELIN FELL

MY GRIEF DIARY

FROM THE AUTHORS

Dear friend,
Thank you for participating in My Grief Diary. I too have suffered from devastating grief, and was looking for a way out. The lessons contained in this workbook proved immensely helpful, and we want to share them with you. Don't be afraid to message me if you have any questions about these assignments, as we are here to help one another. Also, I invite you to join me in both our open and closed groups on Facebook including Grief the Unspoken, National Grief Awareness Day, and Grief Diaries. Grief is a journey that is best walked with others, and we would be honored to have you join us.

With all my love,

Angie Cartwright
Founder, National Grief Awareness Day
angie@nationalgriefawarenessday.com

Dear friend,
Helen Keller once said, "Walking with a friend in the dark is better than walking alone in the light." Moving through grief is one of the hardest challenges we'll ever face and, although each journey is as unique as one's own fingerprint, it's important to know you are not alone in the dark. This workbook is designed to find you in the black abyss of profound sorrow and be your companion along the journey. It offers the very tools we used ourselves to help navigate our own kaleidoscope of emotions, and we are honored to share it with you. May it bring you comfort, healing, and hope.

Warmest regards,

Lynda Cheldelin Fell
Founder, National Grief & Hope Coalition
lynda@lyndafell.com

Important Message to Abuse Victims

If you have experienced sexual abuse, emotional abuse, physical abuse, alcoholism, or drug addiction, you have experienced grief that goes along with it. In your inventory list, you most likely have people who have caused you this pain. When we experience abuse of any kind, we grieve loss of security, loss of normalcy, and loss of trust. We can live in overwhelming fear, and that fear can dominate our other relationships. Naturally, it can be very difficult to write life letters to those who have abused you.

When we forgive someone, it has nothing to do with them. We will never forget nor condone their behavior. It's important that you realize when we can't forgive the person, that person is still hurting you. When we apply our grief inventory to these kinds of relationships, we can start to be free from those who kept us imprisoned. Remember forgiveness is not about condoning their behaviour….it is about freeing yourself.

If you are being abused or suffer from addiction, we suggest you seek professional help. If you need help in finding resources in your area please message us, and we will do our best to get you help. Reading your life letters to your counselor is suggested to provide you with the security you need when doing this.

PART ONE

FACING OUR GRIEF

It's okay to cry. I always feel better after a good cry, like I've released a small bit of the agony. When you're in the middle of the "moment," when you can't stop crying, there is fear that the pain will never end. But allowing yourself those moments are an important part of the healing as we process the deep anguish mixed with the profound love we have for our loved one.

LYNDA CHELDELIN FELL

ASSIGNMENT 1

LISTING OUR GRIEF

DIRECTIONS:
Write down all your losses. If there are more than ten losses, keep writing. Note any memories or thoughts that come up associated with each loss. Please don't rush this. Keep your diary handy and allow yourself some time to keep writing.

LOSS 1 ______________________________

Memory: ______________________________

Thought: ______________________________

____

____

____

LOSS 2 ______________________________

Memory: ______________________________

Thought: ______________________________

____

____

____

LOSS 3 ______________________________

Memory: ______________________________

Thought: ______________________________

____

____

____

One of the first things I realized as I have been on this journey is that I was unaware of all the grief in my heart. If you would have asked me two years ago who I have grieved over, I could have listed my loved ones and my pets. – Angie

Notes, thoughts & doodles:

Grief can be the garden of compassion.

RUMI

LOSS 4 ______________________________

Memory:______________________________

Thought:______________________________

____

____

____

LOSS 5 ______________________________

Memory:______________________________

Thought:______________________________

____

____

____

LOSS 6 ______________________________

Memory:______________________________

Thought:______________________________

____

____

____

LOSS 7 ______________________________

Memory:______________________________

Thought:______________________________

____

____

____

LOSS 8 ______________________________

Memory:______________________________

Thought:______________________________

____

____

____

Notes, thoughts & doodles:

One laugh can scatter a hundred griefs.

LOSS 9 ______________________________

Memory: ______________________________

Thought: ______________________________

____

____

____

LOSS 10 ______________________________

Memory: ______________________________

Thought: ______________________________

____

____

____

More thoughts:

Notes, thoughts & doodles:

A hug is where healing begins.

LYNDA CHELDELIN FELL

ASSIGNMENT 2

WE GRIEVE MANY THINGS

Grief is the normal process of reacting to a loss, any loss. The loss may be physical (such as a death), social (such as divorce), or occupational (such as a job). Now that you have listed your main losses in the last assignment, we want you to look again for more losses in your life. You might not associate them with grief, but grief is usually around when we have these types of losses. Here are other kinds of losses:

- Divorce
- Retirement
- Loss of a relationship
- Fragile health
- Addiction
- Abuse of any kind
- Financial loss
- Empty nest
- Moving
- Spending time in prison
- Having a loved one in prison

DIRECTIONS:
As you did in assignment #1, fully explore your memories around each loss. Write down your thoughts, feelings, and experiences associated with each one. Take your time going through this assignment, do not rush it.

LOSS 11____

Memory:____

Thought:____

LOSS 12____

Memory:____

Thought:____

LOSS 13____

Memory:____

Thought:____

Notes, thoughts & doodles:

It's common to feel that secondary losses pale in comparison to losing a loved one, but the fact remains that we grieve all losses. In the healing process, it's important to validate all the losses we've been through, not just the obvious ones.

LYNDA CHELDELIN FELL

LOSS 14____

Memory:____

Thought:____

LOSS 15____

Memory:____

Thought:____

LOSS 16____

Memory:____

Thought:____

LOSS 17____

Memory:____

Thought:____

LOSS 18____

Memory:____

Thought:____

Notes, thoughts & doodles:

When we treat others with compassion,
we empower their souls.

ANGIE CARTWRIGHT

LOSS 19____________________

Memory:____________________

Thought:____________________

LOSS 20____________________

Memory:____________________

Thought:____________________

At first, I hated the idea of journaling. But when I finally put pen to paper, I unexpectedly found it quite healing and therapeutic. - Lynda

Notes, thoughts & doodles:

Love is the only law capable
of transforming grief into hope.

LYNDA CHELDELIN FELL

ASSIGNMENT 3

THE BIGGER PICTURE

DIRECTIONS:

Combine all losses from assignments #1 and #2 here. We want them all compiled into one list. If you have thought of any more losses, add those too.

1. ______
2. ______
3. ______
4. ______
5. ______
6. ______
7. ______
8. ______
9. ______
10. ______
11. ______
12. ______
13. ______
14. ______
15. ______
16. ______
17. ______
18. ______
19. ______
20. ______

Notes, thoughts & doodles:

Not every day is beautiful,
but there is beauty in every day.

LYNDA CHELDELIN FELL

ASSIGNMENT 4

REACTING TO LOSS

DIRECTIONS:
Answer the following questions.

How do you think your losses have affected you?
Answer: ____________________

Did you ever express the grief you experienced?
Answer: ____________________

How did you handled it?
Answer: ____________________

Have you ever been able to grieve openly about it?
Answer: ____________________

We learn from those around us. I learned that when you are in pain, you drink and you don't talk about it after a while. The adults in my life never handled stress, pain, or problems in a healthy way. They were shown by their parents the same thing. My mother and father could only pass on what had been taught to them. -Angie

Notes, thoughts & doodles:

There is a huge difference between living in the past and remembering the past.

ANGIE CARTWRIGHT

DIRECTIONS:

Write a summary about your losses based upon what you have discovered by completing the last four assignments. What have you discovered so far about you and your life? Please don't rush this. Keep your diary handy and allow yourself some days to keep writing.

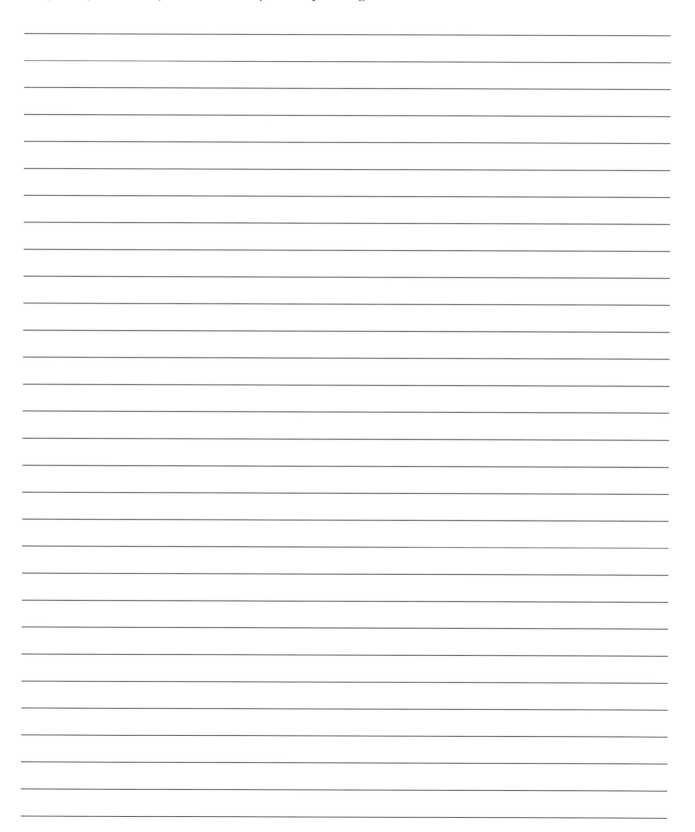

One hello can change a mood.
One hug can change a day.
One hope can change a destiny.

LYNDA CHELDELIN FELL

Compassion can change the world.

ASSIGNMENT 5

REACTING TO PAIN

DIRECTIONS:
List all the ways you reacted to pain in the past. Find a place where you can be alone, a place where you feel safe. It may be your bed, the park, even sitting alone in your car. Shut your phone off. Take several deep breaths. Now look back on your life and **identify how you reacted to pain**.

How did you react to pain in the past? Try to go back as far as you can remember. Please don't rush this. Keep your diary handy and allow yourself some days to keep writing and note any memories or thoughts that come up associated with each pain.

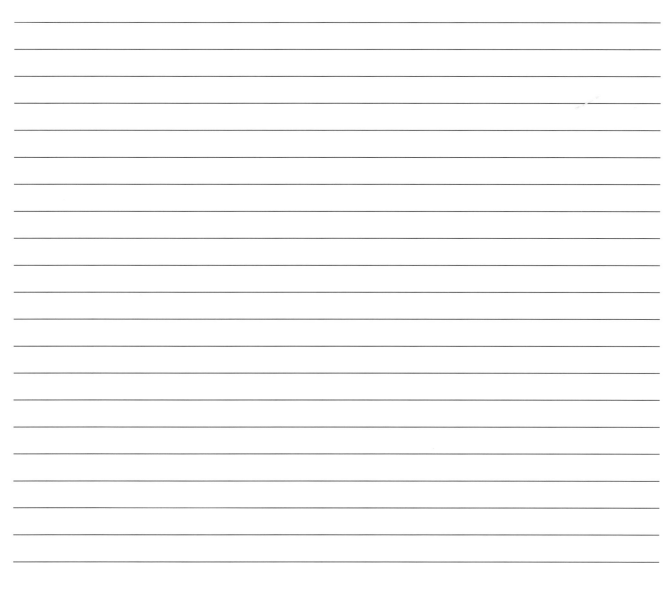

Notes, thoughts & doodles:

Moments are fleeting.
Memories are permanent.
Love is forever.

LYNDA CHELDELIN FELL

ASSIGNMENT 6

FEAR

DIRECTIONS:

List your fears. Take a deep breath and ask yourself the following questions: *What am I afraid of? What scares me? Do I stop myself from healing because I'm afraid?* Take another deep breath, pause for a moment, and then list your fears. Any fear….from spiders to sex. Leave nothing out. No fear is dumb.

FEAR #1: ______________________________

Thoughts associated with this fear:______________________________

____

____

FEAR #2:______________________________

Thoughts associated with this fear:______________________________

____

____

FEAR #3:______________________________

Thoughts associated with this fear:______________________________

____

____

FEAR #4:______________________________

Thoughts associated with this fear:______________________________

____

____

FEAR #5:______________________________

Thoughts associated with this fear:______________________________

____

____

Notes, thoughts & doodles:

What I have discovered in myself is that I have many fears!
Everyone is different, but some of my fears include dying, trying
new things, meeting new people, being accepted, and trusting people.

FEAR #7:____________________

Thoughts associated with this fear:____________________

FEAR #8:____________________

Thoughts associated with this fear:____________________

FEAR #9:____________________

Thoughts associated with this fear:____________________

FEAR #10: ____________________

Thoughts associated with this fear:____________________

Now answer these questions:

Do you let fear run your life? ____________________

Do you act like you are not fearful, but secretly feel paralyzed? ____________________

Are you ready to take your power back and walk through some fear? ____________________

Notes, thoughts & doodles:

Tragedies have a way of waking us up
to what is truly important.

LYNDA CHELDELIN FELL

ASSIGNMENT 7

INVENTORY LIST

DIRECTIONS:

This assignment may be tough, but using your compiled list from Assignment #3, write down everything positive about each event listed, and then write down everything painful about each event listed. This may be difficult with someone who caused you nothing but pain, but try to come up with one positive thing about them. Did they provide you with food or shelter? Did they have a sense of humor? The positive list may be very small for some events, but try. **Below are two examples.**

Loss #1: *My mother died*

Positive (good)
She gave me life
She never physically hurt me
She kept trying
She loved people
She was a good listener

Painful (bad):
Her addiction
She left when I was young
Taking us to foster care

Loss #2: I have fibromyalgia (loss of health)

Positive (good):
It has helped me to be more patient
It has helped me to be more compassionate
It has helped me to slow down and not rush through life

Painful (bad):
I can't do what I use to do
It lowered my self esteem
I am not sexual or even interested

Note: If you start to feel guilty, keep going. Be honest with yourself. Please don't rush this. Keep your diary handy and allow yourself some days to keep writing and note any positive or painful experiences associated with the each loss. Be sure to include the grief you feel for those still living.

Up to this point you have done a lot of work. Congratulate yourself! I believe the hardest work in the world is looking within. By this time in my own workbook, I was able to see how I grieved over so much more than I thought. I also was able to see how I reacted to pain and how much fear there was in most areas of my life.
– Angie

Notes, thoughts & doodles:

Everything looked good on the outside,
but on the inside I was dying.

ANGIE CARTWRIGHT

LOSS 1: ______________________________

Positive: ____________________ Painful: ____________________

Positive: ____________________ Painful: ____________________

Positive: ____________________ Painful: ____________________

Positive: ____________________ Painful: ____________________

LOSS 2: ______________________________

Positive: ____________________ Painful: ____________________

Positive: ____________________ Painful: ____________________

Positive: ____________________ Painful: ____________________

Positive: ____________________ Painful: ____________________

LOSS 3: ______________________________

Positive: ____________________ Painful: ____________________

Positive: ____________________ Painful: ____________________

Positive: ____________________ Painful: ____________________

Positive: ____________________ Painful: ____________________

LOSS 4: ______________________________

Positive: ____________________ Painful: ____________________

Positive: ____________________ Painful: ____________________

Positive: ____________________ Painful: ____________________

Positive: ____________________ Painful: ____________________

Notes, thoughts & doodles:

How to survive grief:
One breath at a time.

LYNDA CHELDELIN FELL

LOSS 5: ______________________________

Positive: ______________ Painful: ______________

Positive: ______________ Painful: ______________

Positive: ______________ Painful: ______________

Positive: ______________ Painful: ______________

LOSS 6: ______________________________

Positive: ______________ Painful: ______________

Positive: ______________ Painful: ______________

Positive: ______________ Painful: ______________

Positive: ______________ Painful: ______________

LOSS 7: ______________________________

Positive: ______________ Painful: ______________

Positive: ______________ Painful: ______________

Positive: ______________ Painful: ______________

Positive: ______________ Painful: ______________

LOSS 8: ______________________________

Positive: ______________ Painful: ______________

Positive: ______________ Painful: ______________

Positive: ______________ Painful: ______________

Positive: ______________ Painful: ______________

Notes, thoughts & doodles:

Grief has nothing to do with a person being strong or weak.

ANGIE CARTWRIGHT

LOSS 9: ____________________

Positive: ____________________ Painful: ____________________

Positive: ____________________ Painful: ____________________

Positive: ____________________ Painful: ____________________

Positive: ____________________ Painful: ____________________

LOSS 10: ____________________

Positive: ____________________ Painful: ____________________

Positive: ____________________ Painful: ____________________

Positive: ____________________ Painful: ____________________

Positive: ____________________ Painful: ____________________

More thoughts:

Notes, thoughts & doodles:

The Ten Rules of Grief
BY LYNDA CHELDELIN FELL

GRIEF RULE #1
There are no rules. Period.

ASSIGNMENT 8

THE TRUE STORY

"Fact Finding" and *"Fact Facing"* is vital to our healing process, to allow ourselves to tell the true story of our loss. Grief can keep us lost in a place where we only tell ourselves the story we believe we can handle because our heart is so broken. As we can see by this point, each loss has both positive and negative aspects. When grieving, we focus *many times on the negative.* But when we do, we often feel guilty. When we remember the good times, we can often feel it is just too much to think about, so we become lost in grief.

For example, Angie shared addiction with her mother:
In 2003, I started the healing process for myself. She joined me years later. After several years we both relapsed. It was one of the saddest times in my life. I went back to sobriety after a few months and she did not. Twenty eight days later she died from a drug overdose. Here are some of the things I told myself after losing her:

- *"I am a horrible daughter. I never helped her. She was always annoying me."*
- *"If I would have went that night she would have been alive today."*
- *"My mother just abandoned me again."*
- *"She just gave up."*
- *"If I wouldn't have relapsed, she would be here today."*

Sound familiar? That's because these thoughts and feelings are normal for grieving people. But how do we find a way out? Society tells us just to not think of those things, yet it is virtually impossible. We are grieving, so it's natural that we continuously try to make sense out of something that doesn't make sense.

DIRECTION:
For each loss listed on your Inventory List, write the thoughts you tell yourself about this relationship or event, whether they are true or false. Please remember to be 100% honest. The more honest you are with yourself, the better you'll feel from these exercises. Then ask yourself this question for each loss listed: What do I feel guilty about with this relationship or loss? Note: Please don't rush this. Keep your diary handy and allow yourself some days to keep writing and note any feelings of guilt or memories associated with each loss.

LOSS #1: ____

My Thoughts: ____

____

____

I feel guilty about this loss because: ______________________________

____

____

Notes, thoughts & doodles:

GRIEF RULE #2

I will grieve my way, not your way.

My way may not make sense to you, but it doesn't make sense to me either.

LOSS #2: ______________________________

My Thoughts: ______________________________

____

____

I feel guilty about this loss because: ______________________________

____

____

LOSS #3: ______________________________

My Thoughts: ______________________________

____

____

I feel guilty about this loss because: ______________________________

____

____

LOSS #4: ______________________________

My Thoughts: ______________________________

____

____

I feel guilty about this loss because: ______________________________

____

____

Notes, thoughts & doodles:

GRIEF RULE #3

The grief timeline is long. If I begin to move on in two months, something is wrong. If I begin to move forward in two years, be impressed.

LOSS #5: ______________________________

My Thoughts: ______________________________

____

____

I feel guilty about this loss because: ______________________________

____

____

LOSS #6: ______________________________

My Thoughts: ______________________________

____

____

I feel guilty about this loss because: ______________________________

____

____

LOSS #7: ______________________________

My Thoughts: ______________________________

____

____

I feel guilty about this loss because: ______________________________

____

____

Notes, thoughts & doodles:

GRIEF RULE #4

Hugs are, and always will be, better than words.

LOSS #8: ______________________________

My Thoughts: ______________________________

____

____

I feel guilty about this loss because: ______________________________

____

____

LOSS #9: ______________________________

My Thoughts: ______________________________

____

____

I feel guilty about this loss because: ______________________________

____

____

LOSS #10: ______________________________

My Thoughts: ______________________________

____

____

I feel guilty about this loss because: ______________________________

____

____

Notes, thoughts & doodles:

GRIEF RULE #5

When you ask me how I am, I will always answer politely.
The truth is too ugly.

ASSIGNMENT 9

ACCEPTING OURSELVES

As we can see from the last assignment, we tell ourselves things that may not be true. Even if they are true, it is necessary to forgive ourselves. We are all human, and there is no one on earth that is perfect.

Go back to the inventory list in assignment #7. Are you now willing to list truthful facts about your relationships and losses? Did you love the person? Did you try to be kind? Did you cause their illness? Please note that these are general questions.

With relationships that were *nothing but bad* (such as physical/sexual abuse), this may be difficult or even impossible to do. You can choose to just move forward at this point or you can privately look to see how you have grown as a stronger, more compassionate, more aware or smarter person because of the event.

Note: If you need to pause and take a deep breath and get a glass of water, this would be a good time to do so. Please don't rush this. Keep your diary handy and allow yourself some days to keep writing and note any truths about the person or loss that come up. There is no right way or wrong way to do this assignment.

When I started doing my grief work, the story that I would tell myself and the inner dialogue started to change for the good! As you learned from my story about my mother in a previous assignment, here are the facts I know today:

- *My mother loved me and told me that, every time she saw me. She showed me love with her actions.*
- *My mother was a grown woman and was able to make her own choices. A few nights before she passed we had a conversation and I told her she needed medical attention. She chose not to go.*
- *My mother tried to make changes in her life throughout her life.*
- *My mother had a disease, she was in pain and wanted to treat her pain. The night she overdosed she was treating her pain. She was powerless over her addiction.*
- *I have helped my mother many times over in her life. I took her into my home many times. I went and picked her up and brought her to town to receive help many times. If she needed something I was always there for her.*

-Angie

Notes, thoughts & doodles:

GRIEF RULE #6

If I question my faith, do not condemn me.
It is normal.

ASSIGNMENT 10

LIFE LETTERS OF EMPOWERMENT

Now it is time to take all the information you have gathered for each loss and put them into Life Letters. These letters can be read by the graveside or at a place that brings you peace. Some find it comforting to imagine the person sitting with you on the couch or across the kitchen table. If it is not possible or you don't like that idea, choose a place that brings you some peace. You also can read your letter to your minister, counselor or caring friend, if you desire.

Please note that your letter may be to someone who is still alive, and we find we're grieving the broken relationship. Maybe you and your siblings are not getting along. It may be over the loss of your parent, or you may not get along with them because of alcoholism. For whatever reason, you have lost that relationship and it can cause our hearts to be broken. We grieve for the relationship to be healed. It may seem weird to write a life letter to someone who is living, but these letters will not be read to them personally. But they are as vital as any other letter.

Here are more ways we grieve the living:

- We have a loved one in prison
- We are adopted and don't know our birth parents
- Our loved one has left for active duty in the services
- We are divorcing

These experiences are just as important as all the others. In time, you may wish to share your letter with them but do not rush this process. It is perfectly ok to imagine them sitting with you and read them the letter or read it to minister, counselor or caring friend.

DIRECTIONS:

Create a Life Letter for each inventory item. Each letter will contain the following parts:

- Forgiveness
- Amends (if needed)
- Thank you
- Closing statement, such as "See you soon," or "Good bye," or "I send you peace."

Letters about other losses such as health, empty nest, moving, etc. are just as vital as the letters to our loved ones. Note: Take your time with each letter. If things change over time from when you write these letters, write one or more new ones anytime you feel the need.

EXAMPLE LETTER #1

Dear Fibro,

I need to write to you to express my feelings. I have a few things I want to say. First of all, I forgive you for taking over my life. I forgive you for the pain you caused in me and my family. I also want to thank you. Since you have arrived in my body, I have learned a lot about myself and how strong I am. You have taught me patience with myself and others. I thank you for teaching me to not judge someone who may not feel good. I have more compassion and understanding than ever before. I am taking my life back. There is more to Angie I have learned, and I thank you for that. I have to go now. Good bye.

Praying for a cure,
Angie

EXAMPLE LETTER #2

Dear Mom,

I needed to write to you to express my feelings about our relationship. When you died there was so much I wanted and needed to tell you. First of all, I wanted to make amends for being so selfish with my time. I know you needed me and I just blew you off. I also am sorry for judging you and your drinking. You really tried hard and I'm so proud of you for that. I'm sorry for being so dominate in our relationship and not allowing you to mother me as you wished.

I forgive you for not being there for me when I was little. I forgive you for the foster homes. I forgive you for not being there for me as a child, I am a parent and have made many mistakes myself.

I wanted to thank you for being patient with me. I thank you for being so kind to your grandchildren and children. Thank you for passing on your beautiful sense of humor and your love for a warm blanket and a cold Pepsi. Thank you for never giving up, you always showed me that we never give up. We may fall but we have to brush ourselves off and keep going. I sure love you and miss you so much. Your legacy will live on through us.

Sending you all the peace in the world, Momma see ya soon!

Love your daughter,
Angie

LIFE LETTER TO LOSS #1

Dear ______________________________,

I am writing you to express my feelings regarding ______________________________

____

____

I forgive you for ______________________________

____

____

____

I want to thank you for ______________________________

____

____

____

In closing, ______________________________

____

____

____

Sincerely – Love – Warm Regards,

____

Your name

____

Notes, thoughts & doodles:

GRIEF RULE #7

Yes, I am blessed to have other children.
But the pain from losing one is worse than agony.

LIFE LETTER TO LOSS #2

Dear ______________________________,

I am writing you to express my feelings regarding ____

____

____

I forgive you for ____

____

____

____

I want to thank you for ____

____

____

____

In closing, ____

____

____

____

Sincerely – Love – Warm Regards,
____

Your name
____

Notes, thoughts & doodles:

GRIEF RULE #8

Consider me a patient of Grief United General.
The first part of my healing begins with a lengthy stay in the ICU.
Please treat me accordingly.

LIFE LETTER TO LOSS #3

Dear ______________________________,

I am writing you to express my feelings regarding ______________________________

____

____

I forgive you for ______________________________

____

____

____

I want to thank you for ______________________________

____

____

____

In closing, ______________________________

____

____

____

Sincerely – Love – Warm Regards,

____

Your name

____

Notes, thoughts & doodles:

GRIEF RULE #9

Do not try to understand my overwhelming emotions.
Your effort will exhaust us both.

LIFE LETTER TO LOSS #4

Dear ______________________________,

I am writing you to express my feelings regarding ______________________________

____

____

I forgive you for ______________________________

____

____

____

I want to thank you for ______________________________

____

____

____

In closing, ______________________________

____

____

____

Sincerely – Love – Warm Regards,

____

Your name

____

Notes, thoughts & doodles:

GRIEF RULE #10

Honor my pain by walking with me.
Not directing me.

LIFE LETTER TO LOSS #5

Dear ______________________________,

I am writing you to express my feelings regarding ____

____

____

I forgive you for ____

____

____

____

I want to thank you for ____

____

____

____

In closing, ____

____

____

____

Sincerely – Love – Warm Regards,

____

Your name

____

Notes, thoughts & doodles:

GRIEF RULE #11

I am not a victim, I am grieving.

Treat my journey with respect and compassion, for your turn will come.

LIFE LETTER TO LOSS #6

Dear ________________________________,

I am writing you to express my feelings regarding ________________________________

____

____

I forgive you for ____

____

____

____

I want to thank you for ____

____

____

____

In closing, ____

____

____

____

Sincerely – Love – Warm Regards,
____

Your name
____

Notes, thoughts & doodles:

GRIEF RULE #12

I know that this is more than the ten rules of grief.
That's because grief doesn't ever make sense.

LIFE LETTER TO LOSS #7

Dear ______________________________,

I am writing you to express my feelings regarding ______________________________

____

____

I forgive you for ______________________________

____

____

____

I want to thank you for ______________________________

____

____

____

In closing, ______________________________

____

____

____

Sincerely – Love – Warm Regards,

____

Your name

____

Notes, thoughts & doodles:

There's a bright future for you at every turn,
even if you miss one.

LIFE LETTER TO LOSS #8

Dear ________________________________,

I am writing you to express my feelings regarding ______________________________

____

____

I forgive you for ____

____

____

____

I want to thank you for ____

____

____

____

In closing, ____

____

____

____

Sincerely – Love – Warm Regards,

____

Your name

____

Notes, thoughts & doodles:

It's easy to hang onto the clothes
if you don't need the hangers.

CAROL SCIBELLI
Author of *Poor Widow Me*

LIFE LETTER TO LOSS #9

Dear ______________________________,

I am writing you to express my feelings regarding ______________________________

____

____

I forgive you for ______________________________

____

____

____

I want to thank you for ______________________________

____

____

____

In closing, ______________________________

____

____

____

Sincerely – Love – Warm Regards,

____

Your name

____

Notes, thoughts & doodles:

No one ever told me that grief
felt so like fear.

C.S. LEWIS

LIFE LETTER TO LOSS #10

Dear ______________________________,
I am writing you to express my feelings regarding ______________________________

____

____

I forgive you for ______________________________

____

____

____

I want to thank you for ______________________________

____

____

____

In closing, ______________________________

____

____

____

Sincerely – Love – Warm Regards,
____

Your name
____

Notes, thoughts & doodles:

When grief is deepest, words are fewest.

ANN VOSKAMP

Congratulations on making it this far!

At this time, you hopefully have discovered some truths about your losses and your grief. By making it this far in the workbook, we hope you begin to experience a shift in the way you see your past, the present, and your future. It may be immediate, or it may develop slowly over a period of time. But now that you have been given some tools, when you find grief tied to any relationship, living or deceased, you can apply these steps to work through it and not become imprisoned by it.

Notes, thoughts & doodles:

There is no pain so great as the memory of joy in present grief.

AESCHYLUS

PART TWO

FACING OUR FUTURE

When we experience a loss, the first feeling for most is that "life is over." This is a normal feeling. The life we once lived **is over,** we are forever changed when we lose something or someone we love. So we must rebuild our lives.

When one is grieving, every moment is crushing, overwhelming, and exhausting. The sadness cloaks every aspect of your life with no offer of escape. How do we not only face the grief, but then walk through it? How do we survive?

Rebuilding isn't done overnight, it is a series of baby steps. In this section of the workbook, we offer you baby steps that build upon each other. Sometimes the baby steps take great effort but, with practice and time, they eventually become easier and then effortless.

Notes, thoughts & doodles:

Hope is patience with the lamp lit.

TERTULLIAN

ASSIGNMENT 11

THE IMPORTANCE OF SELF COMPASSION

In the long days of profound grief, exhaustion sets in easily. Everyday tasks that used to be simple now quickly become overwhelming, which adds to our tears. In addition, our memory inexplicably has deserted us entirely. Even if we muster the energy to tackle an easy household chore, we may forget what we were doing before we even begin. Sound familiar? Whether your answer is yes or no, this is a really important assignment either way....simple, but important.

DIRECTIONS:

Take 5 minutes to think nothing but compassionate thoughts about yourself. Find yourself a quiet spot. It can be your favorite chair, in your car, in your office, or even in your garden. Find a quiet spot, clear your head, and then think nothing but compassionate thoughts about yourself for five minutes. Not your spouse, not your children, not your coworkers, but yourself. Do this every day.

If you're struggling, here are some compassionate thoughts that may apply to you:

I have a ____
Example: good heart, gentle soul, witty personality

I make a ____
Example: good lasagna, potato salad, scrapbook, quilt

I'm a good____
Example: friend, gardener, knitter, painter, poem writer, piano player, volunteer

People would say I'm ____
Example: funny, kind, smart, gentle, generous, patient, humble, good with my hands, creative

People would say I have a ____
Example: good sense of direction, calming voice, good handle on money, cute nose, nice smile

Once you fill in the blanks above, think about each one for a minute or two. Give yourself permission to really validate those positive qualities. Don't be afraid to add things each time you do this assignment.

When I first did this assignment, I struggled. I couldn't fathom any compassionate thoughts about myself, my world had become so very dark and all my thoughts were negative. –Lynda

Notes, thoughts & doodles:

My great hope is to laugh as much as I cry;
to get my work done and
try to love somebody and
have the courage to accept the love in return.

MAYA ANGELOU

ASSIGNMENT 12

TENDER LOVING CARE

While grieving, it is important to consider yourself in the intensive care unit of Grief United Hospital, and treat accordingly. How would the nurses treat you if you were in ICU? They would be compassionate, gentle, and allow for plenty of rest. That is exactly how you should treat yourself.

In addition, soothing sensitive parts of your body with tenderness is an attentive way to honor your emotional pain and, surprisingly, can go a long way toward comforting the whole self. If wearing fuzzy blue socks offers a smidgen of comfort, then wear them unabashedly. If whipped cream on your cocoa offers a morsel of pleasure, then indulge unapologetically. This isn't an excuse for irresponsible or unhealthy behavior. Rather, it's an opportunity to treat our five senses to something soothing....anything that offers a perception of delight. With practice, that awareness of delight will no longer require effort. And, over time, it will help to balance the sadness.

TLC suggestions:

- Shower or bathe with a lovely scented soap
- Soak in a warm tub with Epsom salts and/or a splash of bath oil
- Wear a pair of favorite socks
- Light a fragrant candle
- Listen to relaxing music
- Apply a rich lotion to your skin before bed
- Indulge in a few bites of your favorite treat
- Enjoy a mug of your favorite soothing herbal tea

DIRECTIONS:
List five ways you can offer yourself tender loving care, and then do at least three every day.

TLC #1: ____________________

TLC #2: ____________________

TLC #3: ____________________

TLC #4: ____________________

TLC #5: ____________________

While delighting your senses do nothing to erase the emotional heartache, they do offer a reminder that not all pleasure is forever lost. -Lynda

Notes, thoughts & doodles:

Hope is being able to see that there is light despite all of the darkness.

DESMOND TUTU

ASSIGNMENT 13

SEE THE BEAUTY

Profound grief can appear to rob our world of all beauty. Yet the truth is, and despite our suffering, beauty continues to surround us. The birds continue to sing, flowers continue to bloom, the surf continues to ebb and flow. Reconnecting to our surroundings helps us to reintegrate back into our environment.

Begin by acknowledging one small pleasantry each day. Perhaps your ears register the sound of singing birds. Or you catch the faint scent of cookies baking in a neighbor's kitchen. Or notice the sun's illumination of a nearby red rosebush. Give yourself permission to notice one pleasantry, and allow it to really register within your body and soul. Here are some suggestions:

- Hear the birds sing
- Observe some pretty cloud formations
- Visit a nearby park and listen to the children laughing
- Notice the pretty colors of blooming flowers
- Sit on a beach or at the edge of a lake
- Search for interesting rocks
- Attend a local concert, play, or comedy act
- Hike a popular trail

DIRECTIONS:
List five ways you can observe the beauty around you, and then try to accomplish at least three every day.

BEAUTY #1: ____________________

BEAUTY #2: ____________________

BEAUTY #3: ____________________

BEAUTY #4: ____________________

BEAUTY #5: ____________________

Listening to the birds outside my bedroom window every morning was something I had loved since childhood. But when Aly died I found myself deaf and blind to the beauty around me, like I had become part of a strange movie, colorless and silent. On one particular morning as I fought the urge to stay in bed, I halfheartedly noticed the birds chirping outside my bedroom window. My heart sank as I realized that they had been chirping all along, but I was now deaf to their morning melody. Panic set in as I concluded that, without my daughter, I would never enjoy the beauty in life ever again. Briefly entertaining suicide to escape the profound pain, I quickly ruled it out. My family had been through so much already, I couldn't add to their profound sorrow. But by making the choice to live, I had to find a way to allow beauty back into my life. So on that particular morning as I lay in bed, I forced myself to listen and really hear the birds. Every morning from that point forward, I repeated that same exercise. With persistent practice, it became easier and then eventually effortless to appreciate the birds' chirping and singsongs once again. My world is now full of beautiful color and glorious sounds, and not devoid of all beauty like I had feared. -Lynda

Notes, thoughts & doodles:

There is no medicine like hope.

ORISON SWETT MARDEN

ASSIGNMENT 14

PROTECT YOUR HEALTH

Studies show that profound grief throws our body into "flight or fight" syndrome for months and months. This prolonged physiological response can often cause physical unbalance resulting in compromised immunity and illnesses. Thus it becomes critical to guard our physical health.

Resist the urge to seek refuge in damaging substances such as alcohol or illicit drugs. Instead, nourish your body by way of healthful eating, small amounts of light exercise such as walking the dog or with a friend, and doing your best to practice good sleep hygiene.

A stronger physical health can help anchor us in times of emotional upheaval. Opportunities to help protect our health:

- Practice good sleep hygiene
- Drink plenty of water
- Take a short walk, or other form of exercise, outside every day
- Limit simple carbohydrates
- Keep a light calendar and guard your time carefully, don't allow others to dictate and overflow your schedule
- If your diet isn't balanced, incorporate one healthful addition daily, such as a protein shake, fiber bar, or handful of dried blueberries

DIRECTIONS:
List five ways you can improve your health. And then ensure you incorporate at least three into your day, every day.

STEP #1: ____________________

STEP #2: ____________________

STEP #3: ____________________

STEP #4: ____________________

STEP #5: ____________________

After our daughter's accident I soon found myself fighting an assortment of viruses including head colds, stomach flus, sore throats and more, compounding my already frazzled emotions. It was then that I realized how far reaching the effects of grief has, that it truly touches every part of our life including our physical health. -Lynda

Notes, thoughts & doodles:

There are two ways of spreading light:
to be the candle or the mirror that reflects it.

EDITH WHARTON

ASSIGNMENT 15

FIND AN OUTLET

For a long time in the grief journey, everything is painful. In the early days, just getting out of bed and taking a shower can be exhausting. Housecleaning, grocery shopping, and routine appointments often take a backseat or disappear altogether. As painful as it is, it's very important to find an outlet that gets you out of bed each day. Finding something to distract you from the pain, occupy your mind, and soothe your senses can be tricky, but possible. And performing a repetitive act can soothe your physical senses and calm your mood, and even result in a new craft or gifts your family and friends will treasure.

Although a new outlet may feel exhausting at first, this step is critical to your future well-being. It doesn't mean you have to do it forever, just focus on it for the time being. Possible activities include:

- Learn to mold chocolate
- Learn to create soap
- Learn how to knit, crochet, or quilt
- Make something from your loved one's clothing
- Take up beading
- Learn a new sport such as golf or kayaking
- Create a memorial garden
- Join Pinterest
- Join a book club
- Renovate one room
- Volunteer at a local shelter
- Sign up for an enrichment class

DIRECTIONS:
List five possible outlets. And then take steps to start at least one.

OUTLET #1: ______________________________

OUTLET #2: ______________________________

OUTLET #3: ______________________________

OUTLET #4: ______________________________

OUTLET #5: ______________________________

Three months after our daughter's accident, my dear husband and I sought refuge in a quaint little town on a nearby island. While browsing through the boutiques with a heavy heart, I stopped to admire a basket of highly fragrant soaps. On a whim, I decided to teach myself how to make soap and soon discovered that the soothing action of stirring a pot of fragrant ingredients proved to be very therapeutic. Thus, making Tear Soap became my outlet for many months. -Lynda

Notes, thoughts & doodles:

How wonderful to be able to let go
and smile again, long before you die.

CAROL SCIBELLI

ASSIGNMENT 16

THE FUTURE

DIRECTIONS:
List five small goals you would like to achieve in the next year.

GOAL #1:____

GOAL #2:____

GOAL #3:____

GOAL #4:____

GOAL #5:____

Look hard at your goals. Is anything standing in your way of achieving them? If so, list the obstacles here.

Obstacle #1: ____

Obstacle #2: ____

Obstacle #3: ____

Obstacle #4: ____

Obstacle #5: ____

Obstacle #6: ____

Obstacle #7: ____

Obstacle #8: ____

Obstacle #9: ____

Obstacle #10: _______________________________________

For any goal with an obstacle, re-word or revise that goal here.

GOAL #1:____

GOAL #2:____

GOAL #3:____

GOAL #4:____

GOAL #5:____

Notes, thoughts & doodles:

Once you choose hope,
anything is possible.

CHRISTOPHER REEVE

Now, list the steps needed to accomplish each goal.

EXAMPLE:
Goal: Write a book about my loss
Step 1: Decide what I want to tell people, and why. Can I help others?
Step 2: Decide on a title
Step 3: Research options for getting my book published
Step 4: Start writing 30 minutes every day

GOAL #1: ____________________

Step 1: ____________________

Step 2: ____________________

Step 3: ____________________

GOAL #2: ____________________

Step 1: ____________________

Step 2: ____________________

Step 3: ____________________

GOAL #3: ____________________

Step 1: ____________________

Step 2: ____________________

Step 3: ____________________

GOAL #4: ____________________

Step 1: ____________________

Step 2: ____________________

Step 3: ____________________

GOAL #5: ____________________

Step 1: ____________________

Step 2: ____________________

Step 3: ____________________

Notes, thoughts & doodles:

Let your hopes, not your hurts shape your future.

ROBERT H. SCHULLER

Dear friend,

The baby steps offered in Part 2 of this workbook are just that....baby steps. While they don't erase or invalidate the pain, the truth is that if you treat yourself kindly, allow yourself small measures of comfort, and find a healthy outlet for your grief, you'll feel better. And if you feel better, you'll cope better. These steps can not only help bring comfort, but they can also offer focus and purpose, a light in the darkness, until you find the sunshine once again.

This brings us to the end of the workbook, and a new beginning for the life ahead. It may not be the same life you had, but it is a life worth living and with time and patience, your grief dance will eventually turn into solid footing, which will lead to purposeful steps toward finding moments of peace and joy.

But remember, no matter where you are on your journey, we are always right beside you.

With all our love,

Lynda Cheldelin Fell
& Angie Cartwright

Notes, thoughts & doodles:

The beautiful thing about hope
is that it has no expiration date.

LYNDA CHELDELIN FELL

RESOURCES

WEBSITES

Lynda Cheldelin Fell	www.lyndafell.com
Angie Cartwright	www.angiecartwright.org
Grief Diaries	www.griefdiaries.com
National Grief Awareness Day	www.nationalgriefawarenessday.com
Good Grief Worldwide	www.goodgriefww.com
National Grief & Hope Coalition	www.helphealhope.org

FACEBOOK PAGES

Grief the Unspoken	www.facebook.com/grieftheunspoken
Grief Diaries	www.facebook.com/GriefDiaries
National Grief Awareness Day	www.facebook.com/nationalgriefawarenessday
National Grief & Hope Convention	www.facebook.com/griefconvention
National Grief & Hope Coalition	www.facebook.com/helphealhope
Angie Cartwright, Public Figure	www.facebook.com/AngieCartwrightGrief
Lynda Cheldelin Fell, Public Figure	www.facebook.com/PowerofOneMoment

FACEBOOK GROUPS

CLOSED GROUPS (must ask permission to join; your posts are not visible to others outside the group)

Grief the Unspoken (GTU)	www.facebook.com/groups/griefunspoken
GTU - Grief Diaries	www.facebook.com/groups/475881435879735
GTU – Grieving Parents	www.facebook.com/groups/390815157638000
GTU – For Widows & Widowers	www.facebook.com/groups/237646546348711
GTU - Teens & Young Adults	www.facebook.com/groups/1426561724289547
GTU – Losing a Loved One to Overdose	www.facebook.com/groups/747482248681795
GTU – Candle Lighting Sanctuary	www.facebook.com/groups/1740885262803429
GTU – Prayer Room	www.facebook.com/groups/1427845387490663
GTU – Loss of a Grandparent	www.facebook.com/groups/136117183192229
GTU – Loss of a Sibling	www.facebook.com/groups/247647045348572
GTU – Loss of a Parent	www.facebook.com/groups/291760674249800
GTU – Pictures of Our Loved Ones	www.facebook.com/groups/465635070121695
GTU – Loss of fiancé, boyfriend/girlfriend	www.facebook.com/groups/158013434372416
GTU – Loss by suicide	www.facebook.com/groups/193304607475819
GTU – Venting, Screaming & Cursing Grief	www.facebook.com/groups/334595596639207

BLOGS

Confessions of a Grieving Mother	www.astrokeoflove.blogspot.com
Grief Diaries Uncensored	www.griefdiariesuncensored.blogspot.com

Notes, thoughts & doodles:

In helping others, we help ourselves.

LYNDA CHELDELIN FELL

ABOUT

LYNDA CHELDELIN FELL

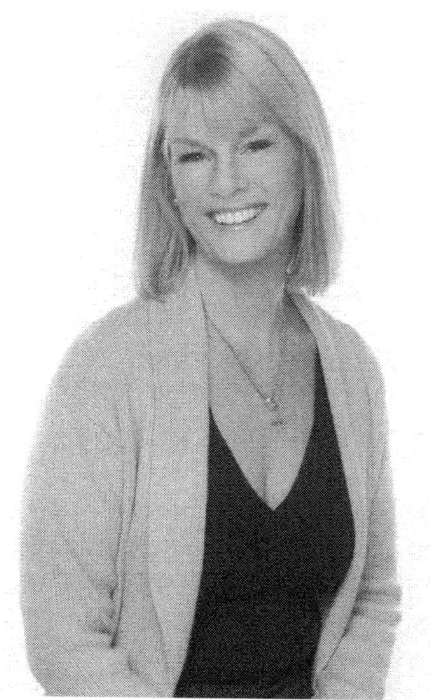

Lynda Cheldelin Fell is an inspirational visionary and entrepreneur who found herself beginning the long journey through profound grief when her 15 year-old daughter died in a car accident in 2009. Two years later, Lynda's world took another unexpected turn two years later when her 46 year-old husband suffered a major stroke leaving him with permanent disabilities, leaving her with a new layer of grief.

Through the darkness, Lynda found comfort by helping others who were struggling, and this fueled her passion to create a legacy of light for the hurting, ignored, and forgotten. She founded AlyBlue Media, in memory of her beloved daughter, to house her growing endeavors that now take her across the country.

Lynda is board president of the National Grief & Hope Coalition, creator of Grief Diaries brand of books, radio, film, and webinars, a post tragedy community facilitator, international bestselling author, member of TheBlaze Branded Contributor Network. She owns AlyBlue Media and is passionate about creating projects focusing on validation, bits of wisdom, and hope.

Contact Lynda:

Twitter:	@lyndafell
Web:	www.lyndafell.com
Email:	lynda@lyndafell.com
FB:	FB/PowerOfOneMoment
Blog:	http://astrokeoflove.blogspot.com/
IMDb:	www.imdb.com/name/nm6837604/
Google+:	plus.google.com/+LyndaCheldelinFell
LinkedIn:	www.linkedin.com/in/lyndacheldelinfell
TheBlaze:	www.theblaze.com/author/lynda-cheldelin-fell/
Amazon:	www.amazon.com/Lynda-Fell/e/B00H2DTRAM
GoodReads:	www.goodreads.com/author/show/7541046.Lynda_Cheldelin_Fell
iTunes:	itunes.apple.com/us/podcast/grief-diaries-radio-show/id850546080?mt=2

ABOUT

ANGIE CARTWRIGHT

Angie Cartwright is the founder of National Grief Awareness Day, occurring on August 30 of each year. She is also the co-founder of We Care Grief Support. Angie has experienced the pain of loss many times in her life starting with the loss of her baby sister when Angie was just 5 years old, the loss of Angie's newlywed husband from a tragic car accident at the tender age of 21, and the loss of her mother from an accidental overdose. Learning the hard way that grievers are often misunderstood, Angie is committed to help change how our culture understands and views grief. She expertly coaches and comforts people all around the world through social media, her website, and her Grief Release Course, to help them find solid footing once again. "I finally realized there was only one thing I could ever do to be free," shares Angie. "It was to embrace my humanness."

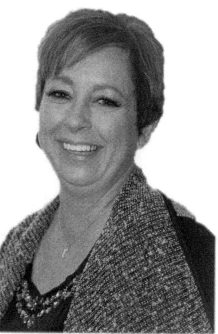

Contact Angie:
Twitter: @TheGTU
Web: www.angiecartwright.org
Email: angie@nationalgriefawarenessday.org
FB: FB/AngieCartwrightGrief
Blog: www.griefdiariesuncensored.blogspot.com
Google+: plus.google.com/+AngieCartwright
LinkedIn: https://www.linkedin.com/in/angiecartwrightgrief
iTunes: itunes.apple.com/us/podcast/grief-diaries-radio-show/id850546080?mt=2

It's important that we share our experiences with other people.
Your story will heal you, and your story will heal somebody else.
When you tell your story, you free yourself and give other
people permission to acknowledge their own story.
IYANLA VANZANT

*

Published by AlyBlue Media
Inside every human is a story worth sharing.
www.AlyBlueMedia.com

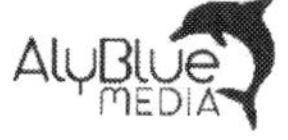